This book is dedicated to my students.
-Mrs. Dorcely

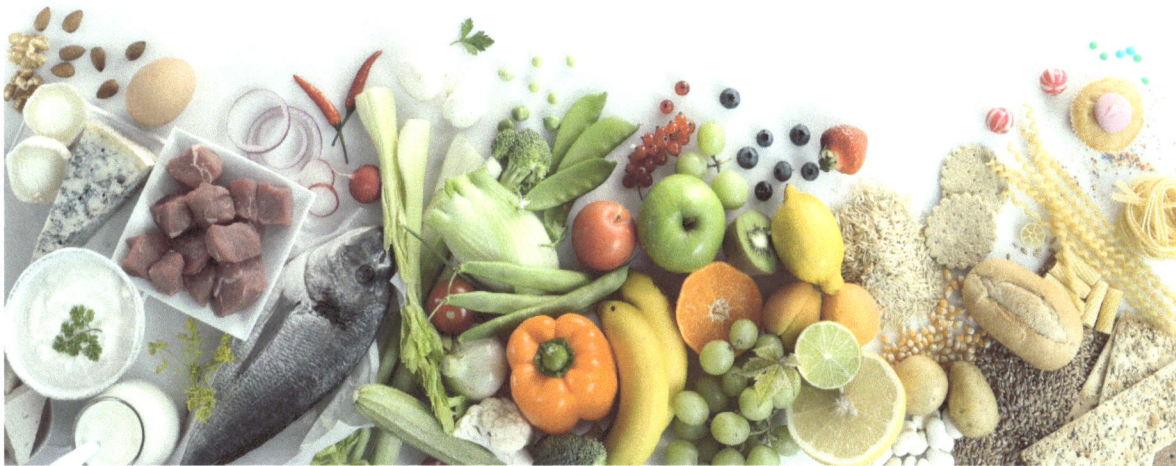

This book belongs to:

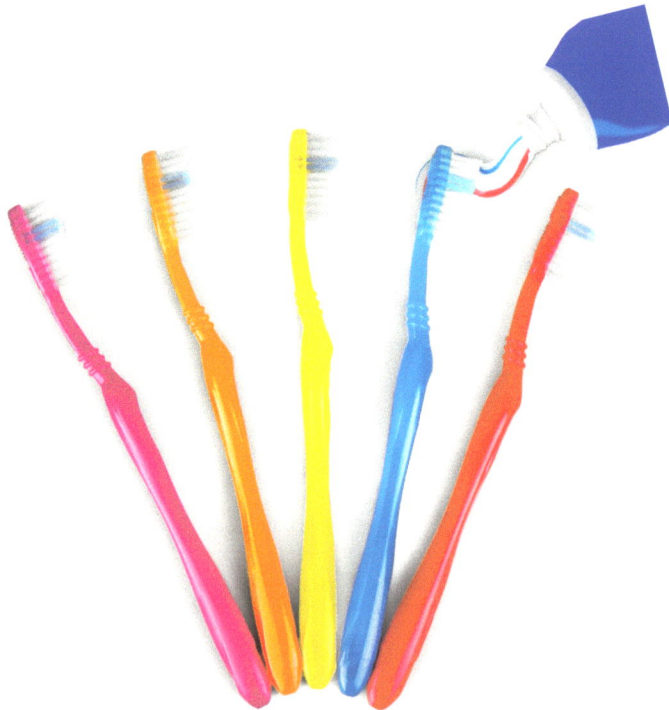

_____

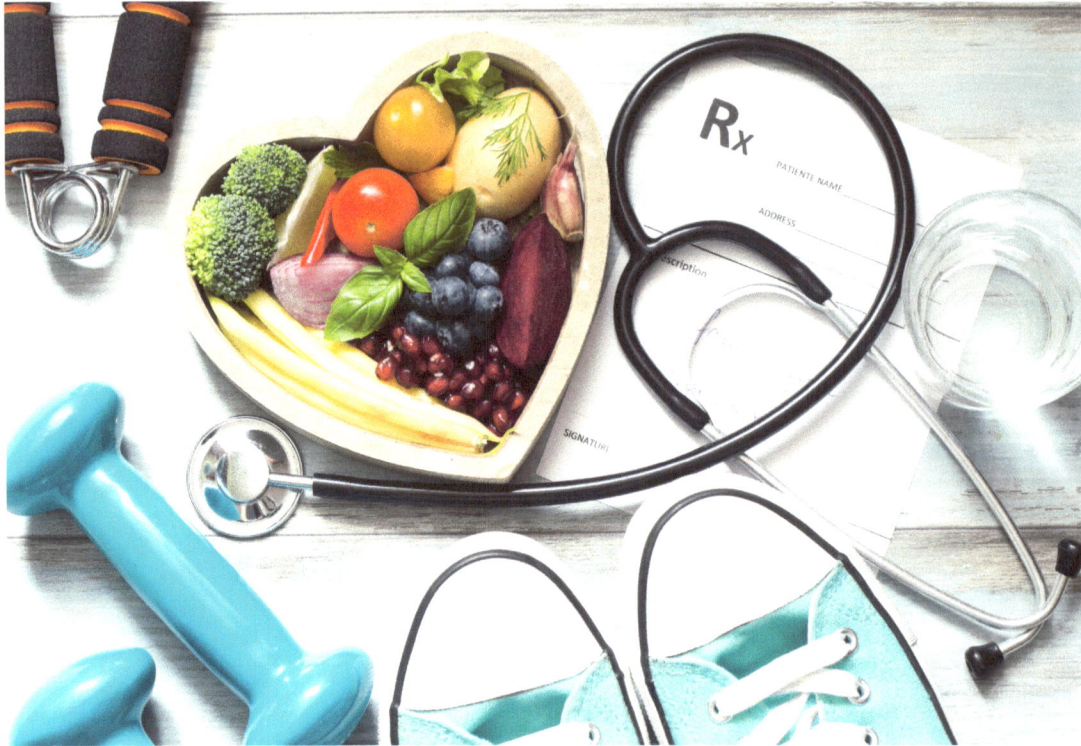

Ms. K says, "This month we are going to learn about ways to stay healthy."

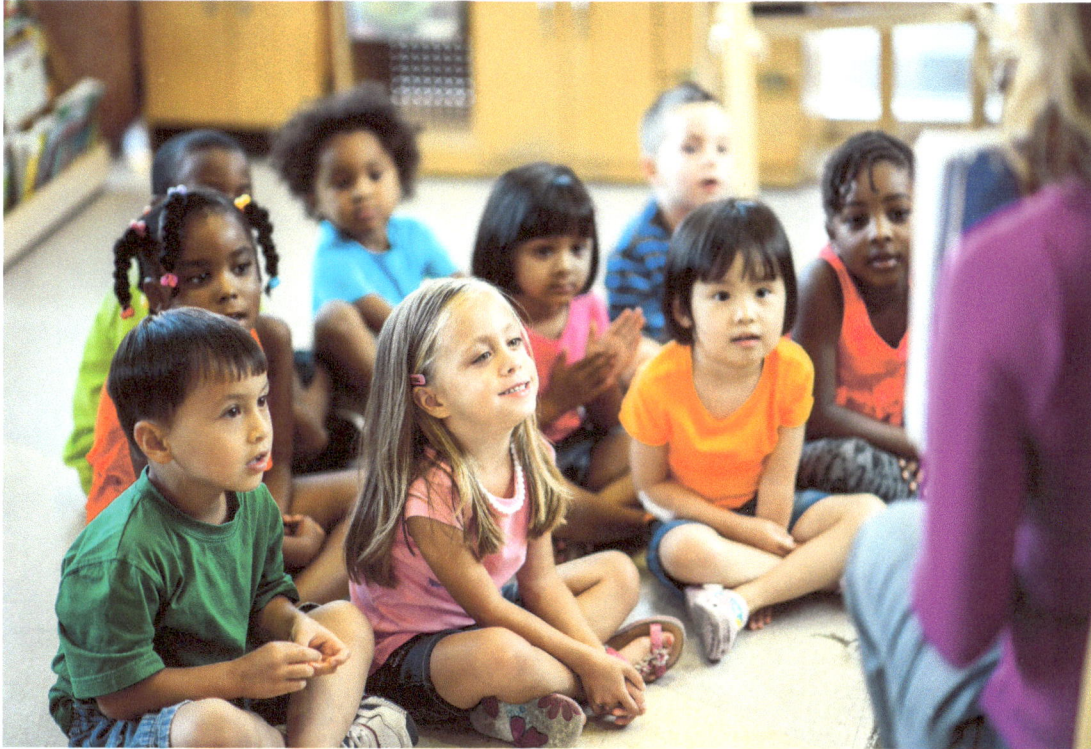

**She asks the children,
"How do you stay healthy?"**

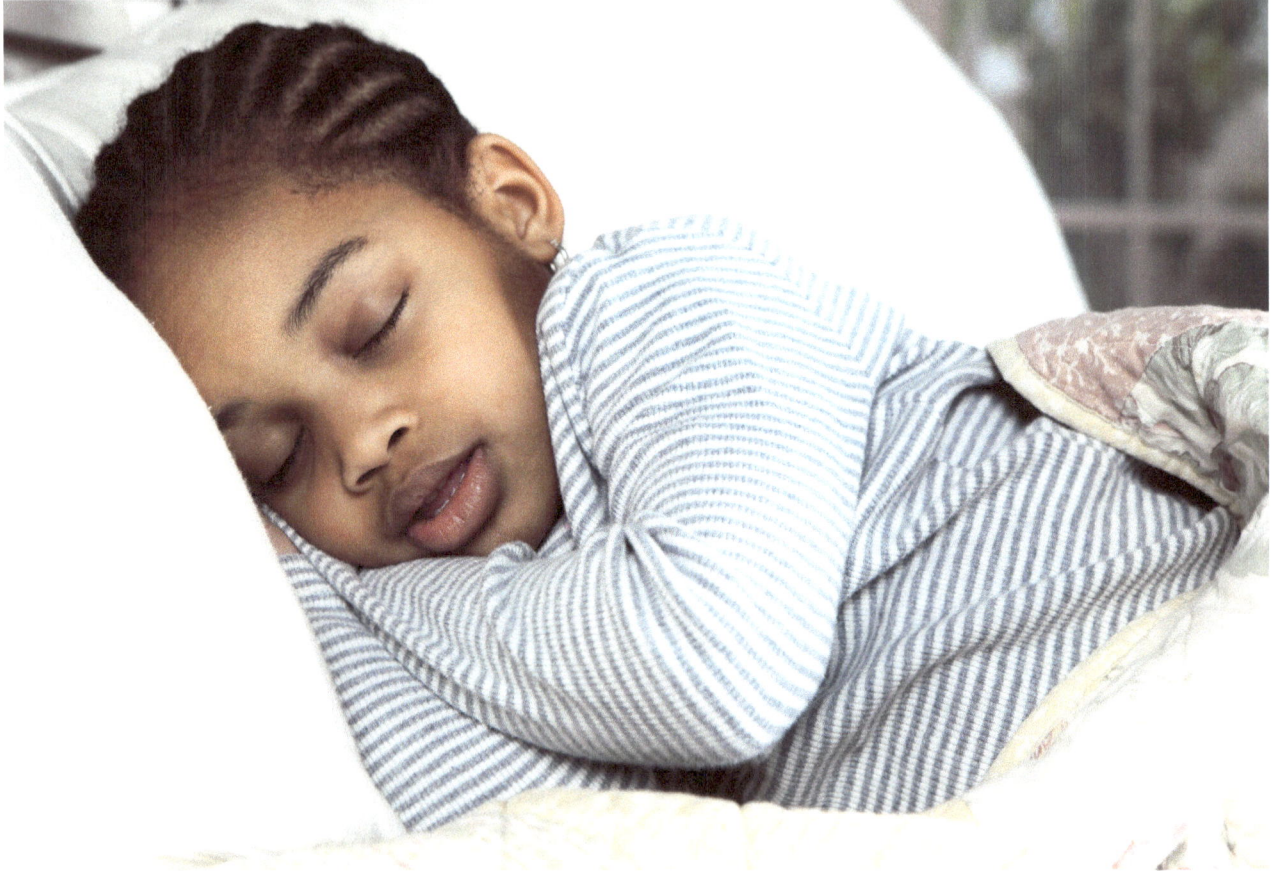

Some children say,
"We have to sleep 8 to 10 hours every night."

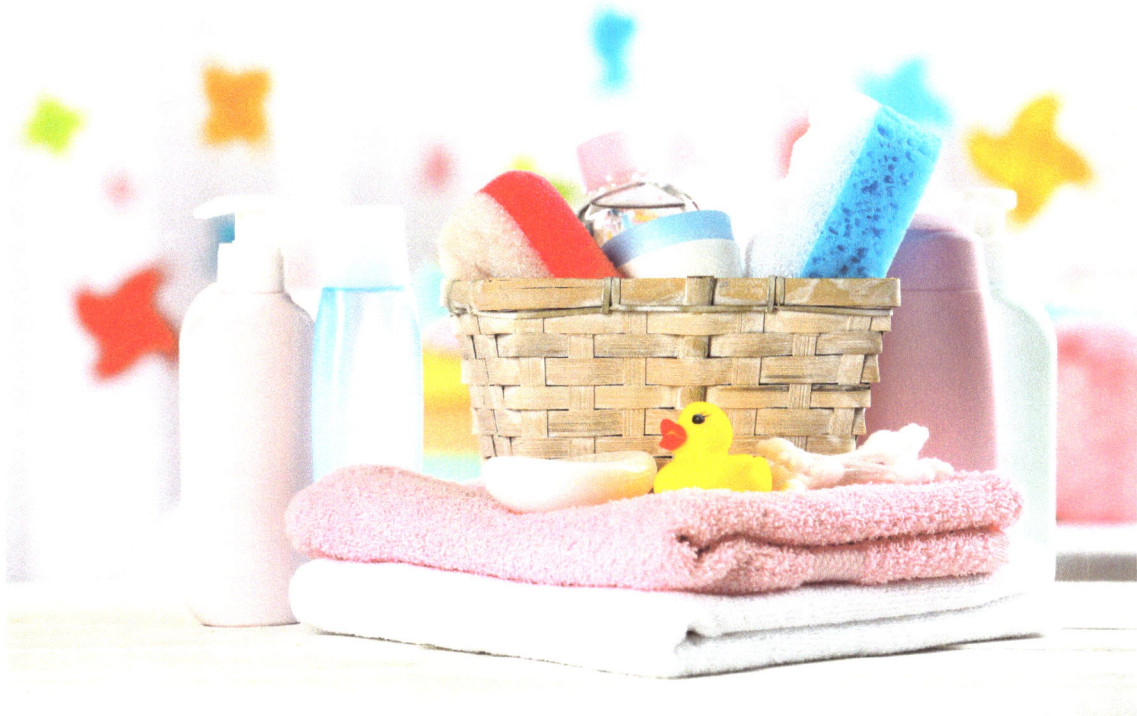

**Some children say,
"We need to have clean bodies
to stay healthy."**

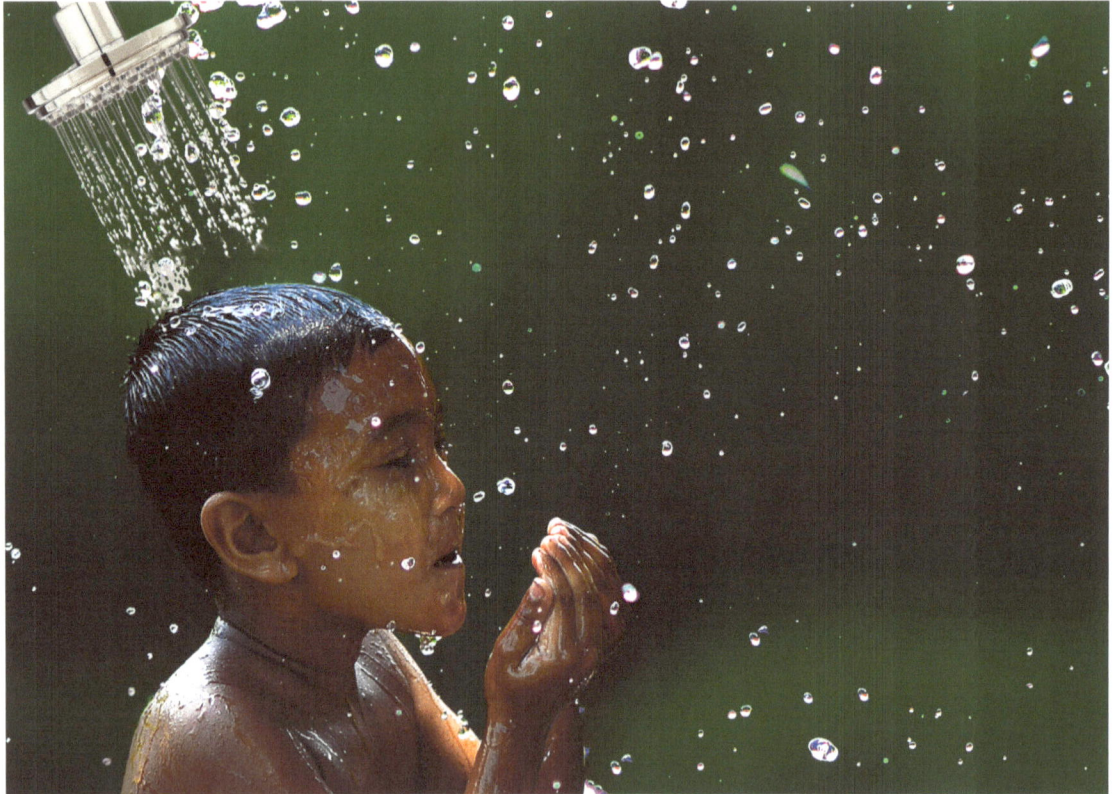

We have to take a shower.

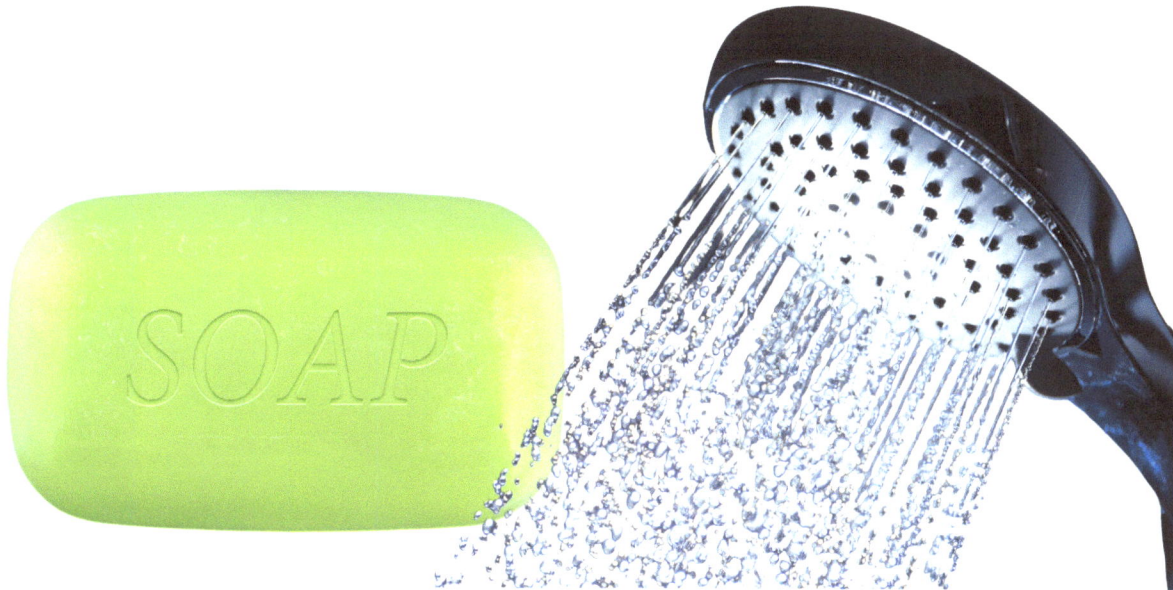

We take a shower with soap and water.

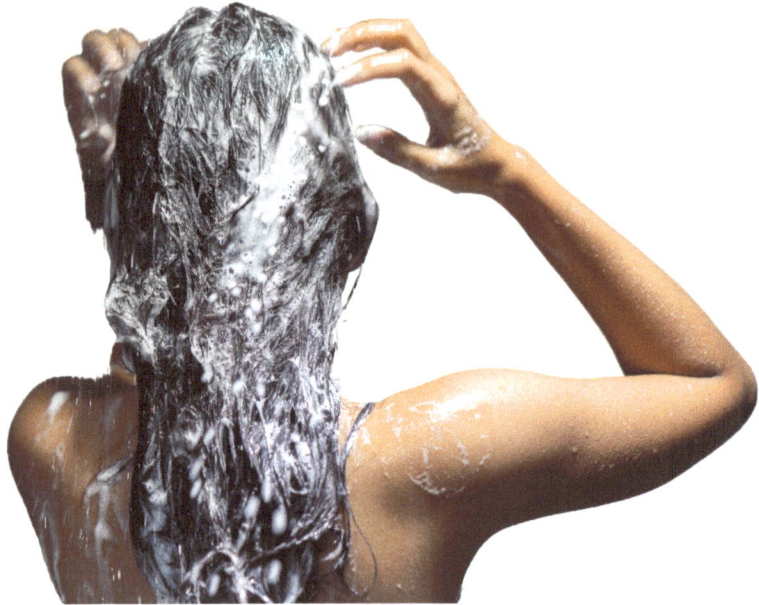

We have to wash our hair.

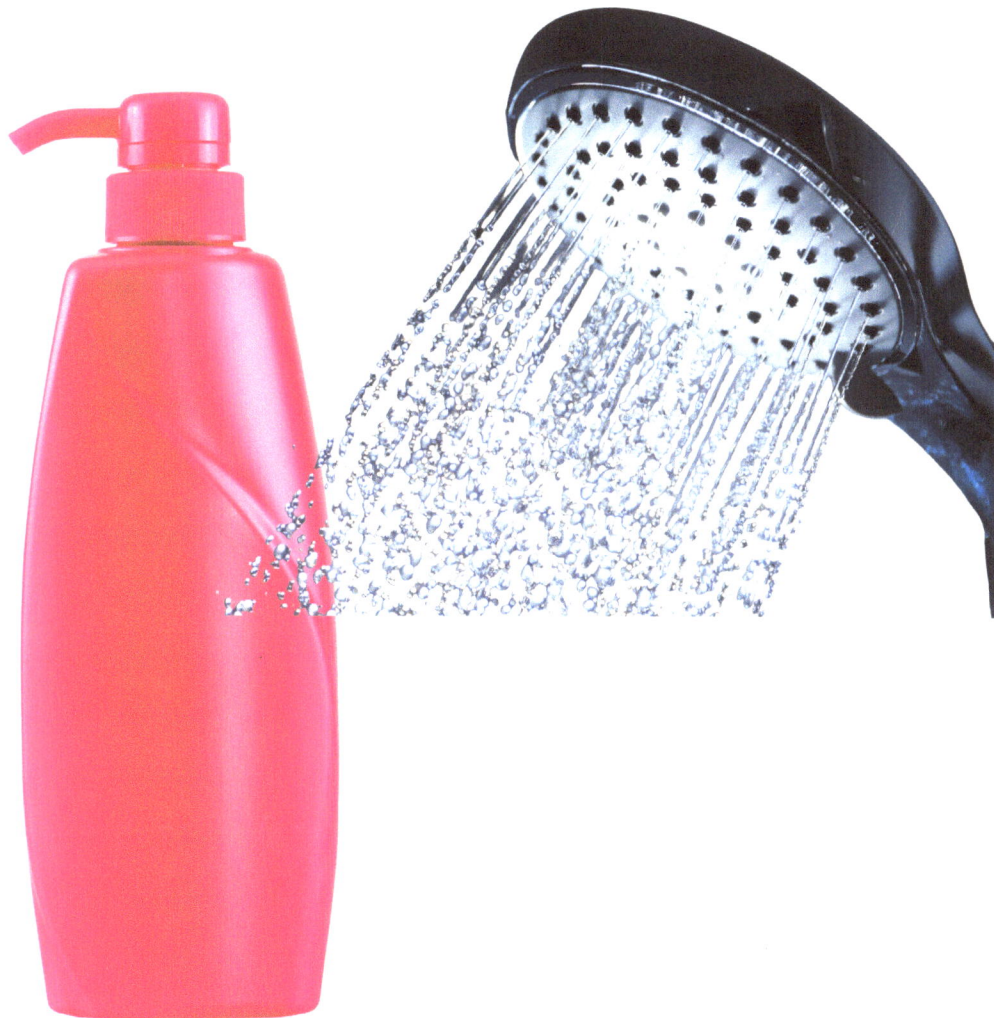

We wash our hair with shampoo and water.

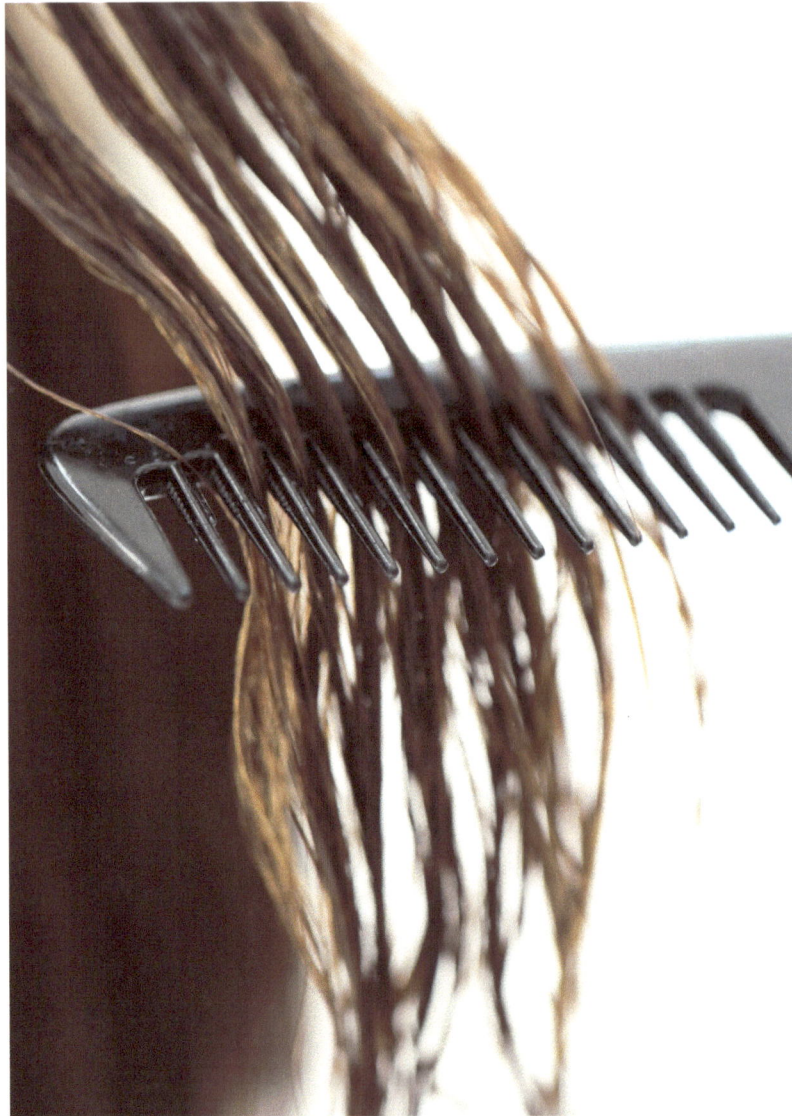

We comb our hair.

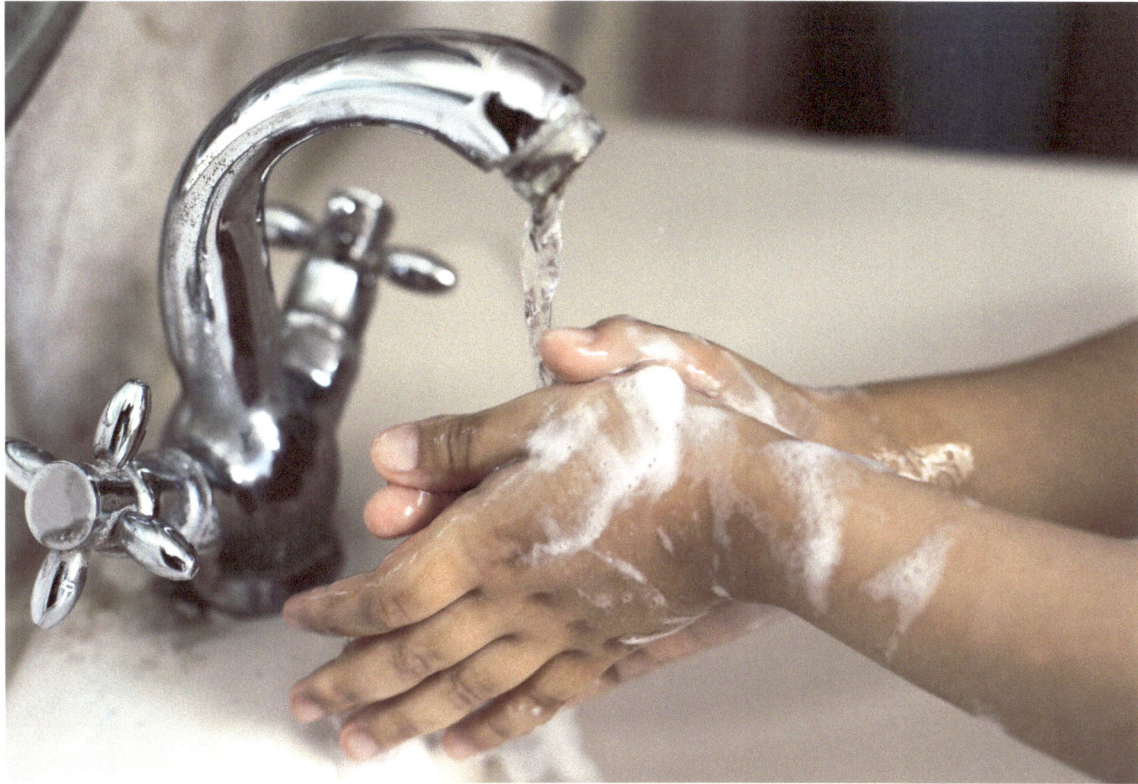

We have to wash our hands to stay healthy.

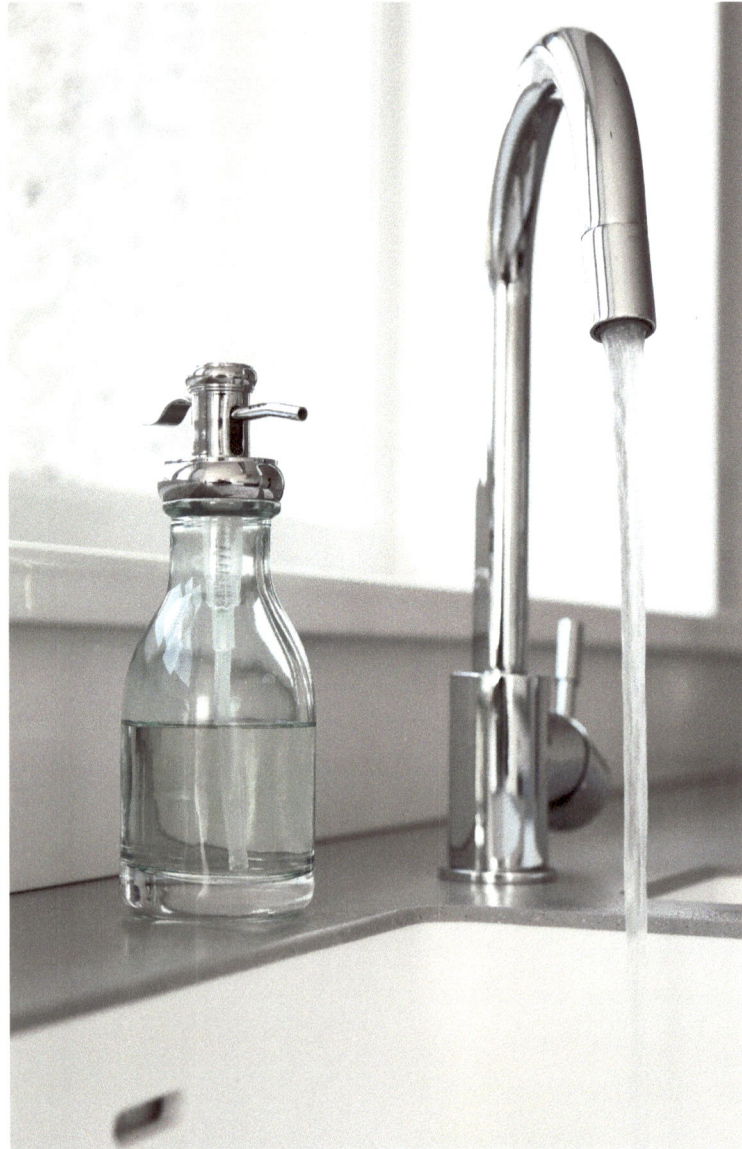

We wash our hands with soap and water.

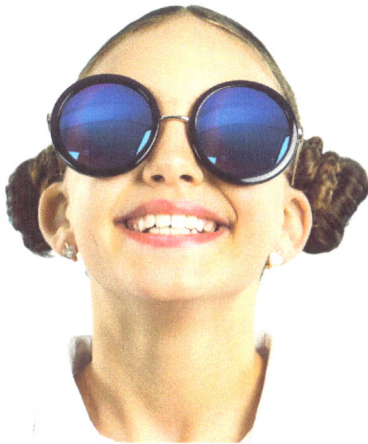

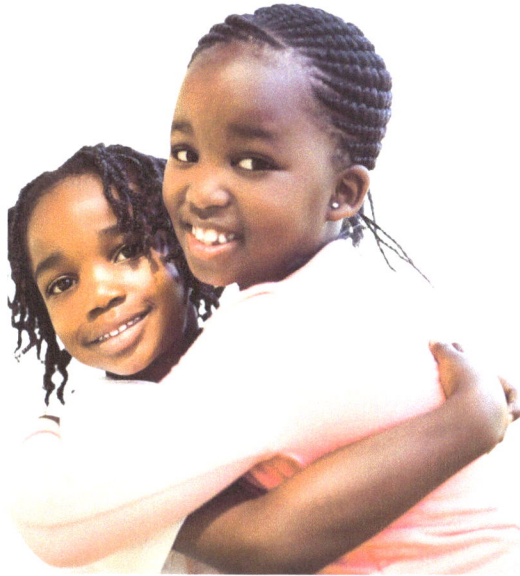

**Some children say,
"We need to have clean teeth to stay healthy."**

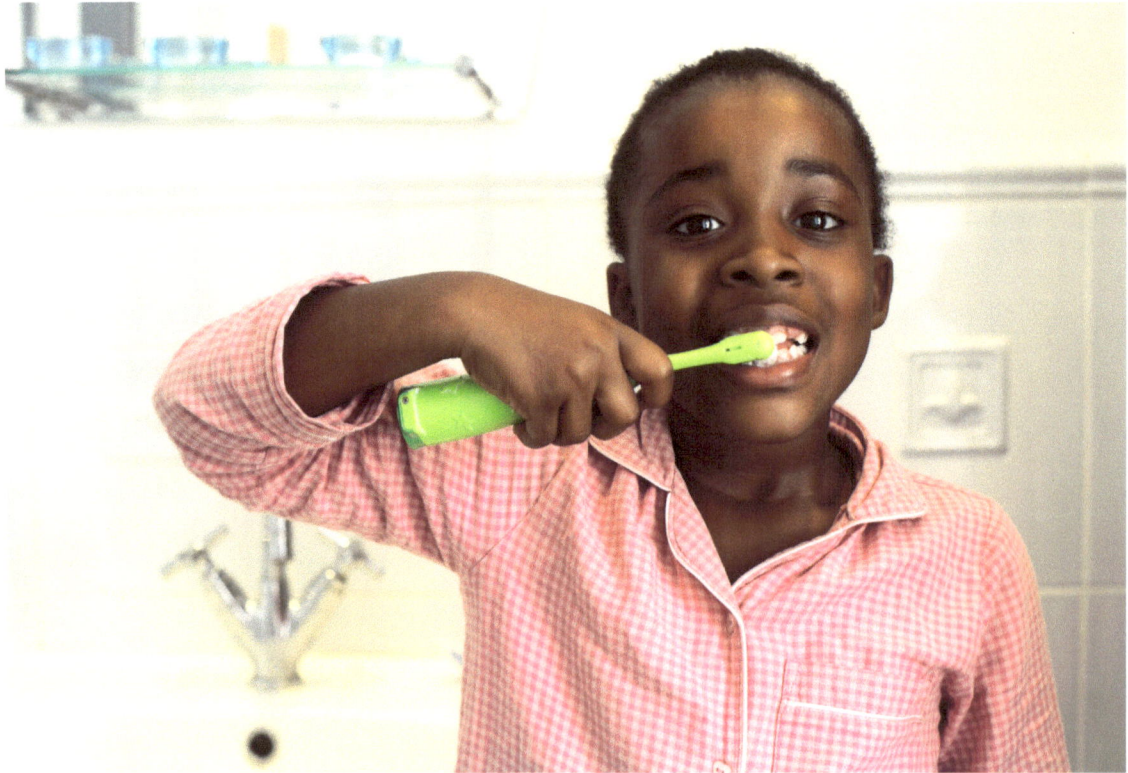

We have to brush our teeth.

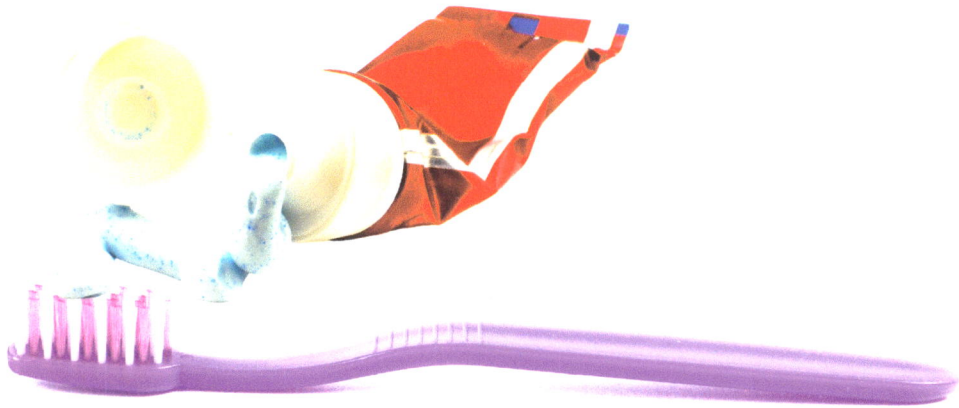

We brush our teeth with a toothbrush and toothpaste.

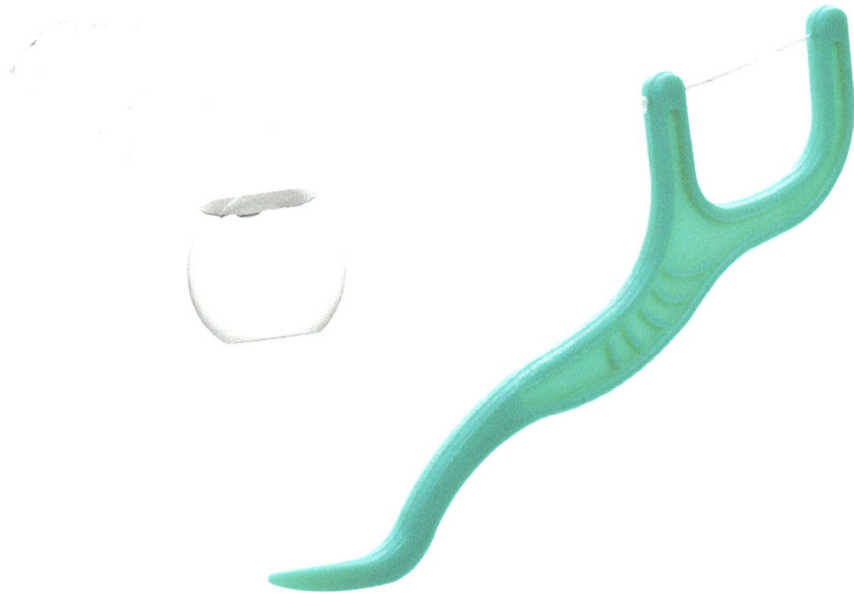

We have to floss our teeth.

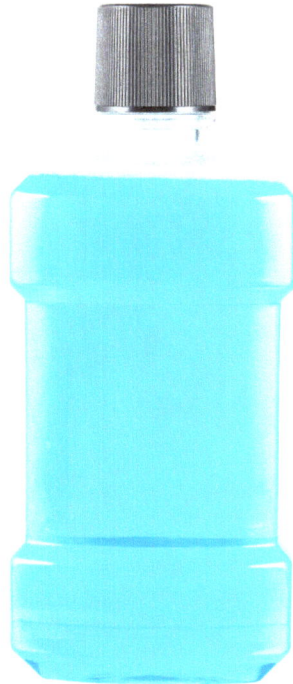

We rinse out our mouth with mouthwash .

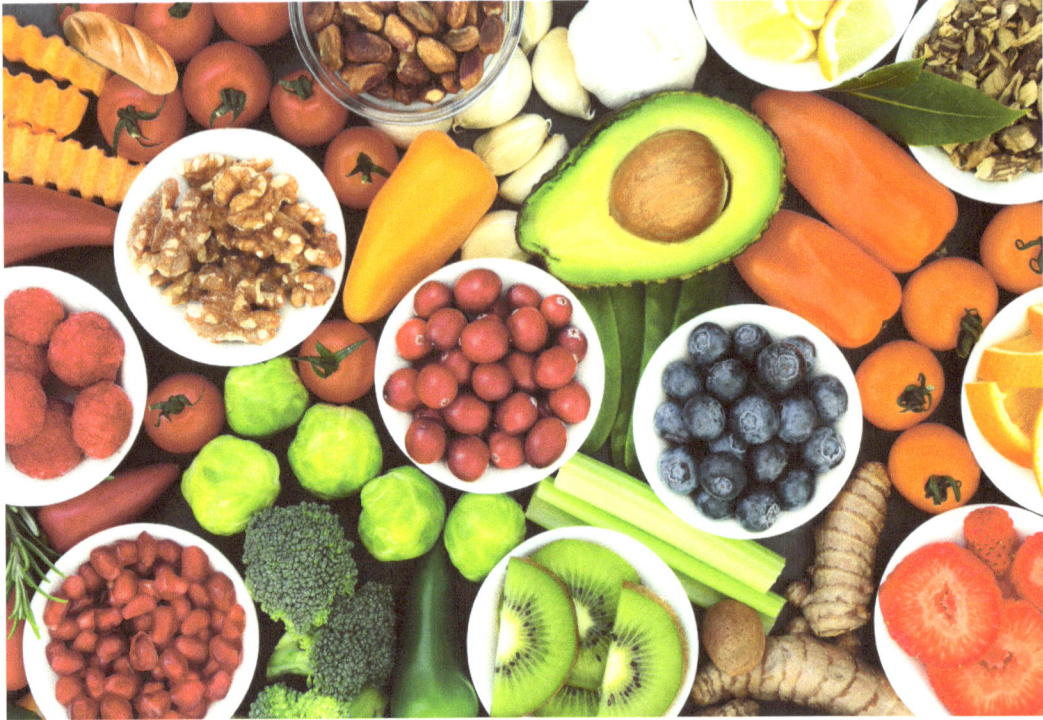

Some children say,
"We have to eat healthy food to stay healthy."

Vegetables

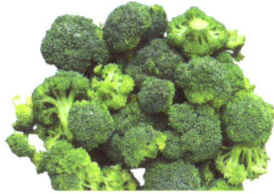

Protein

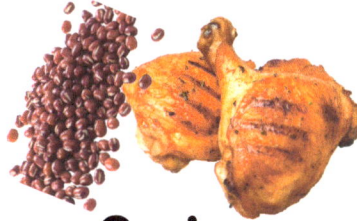

Fruits

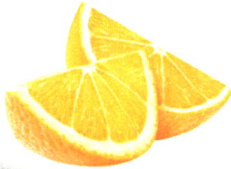

Grain

Dairy

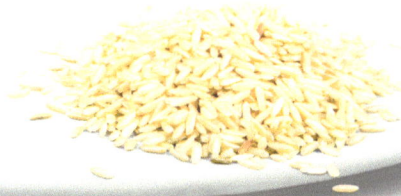

Look at our plate!
We eat a balanced meal.

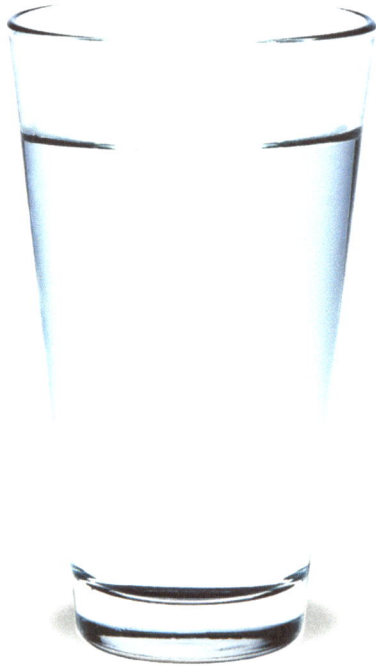

We have to drink water.

What is on your plate?
It's your turn to make a balanced meal!

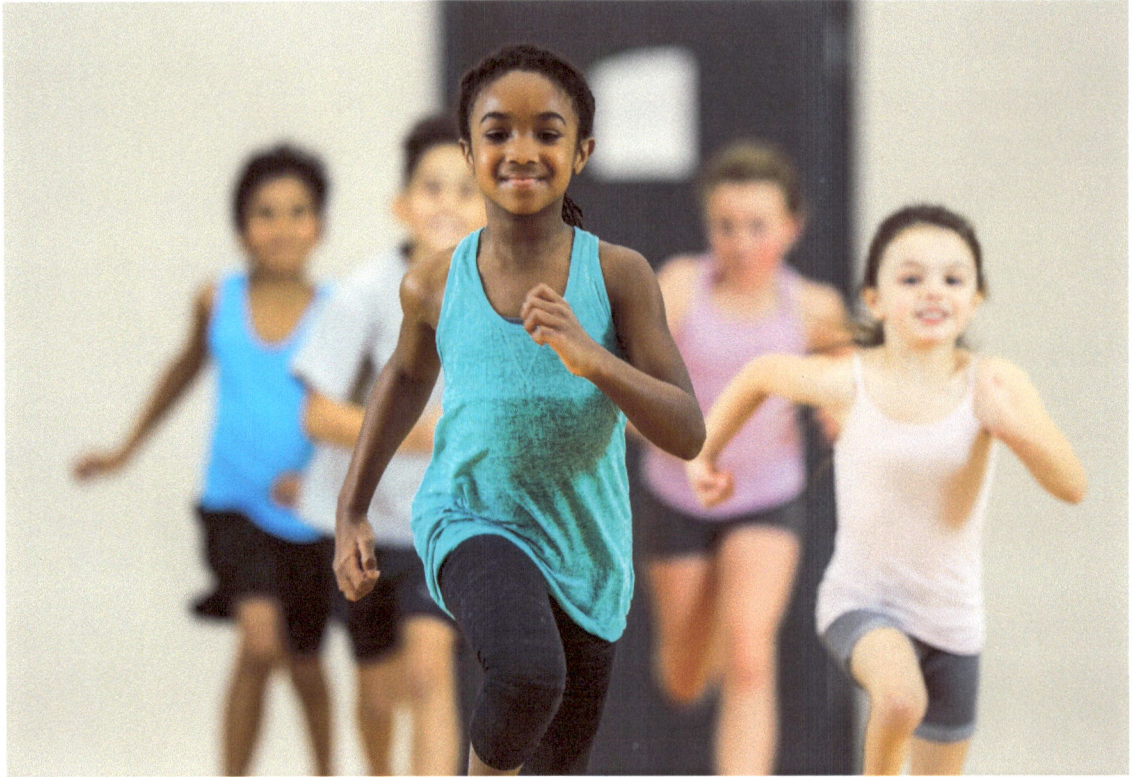

Some children say,
"We have to exercise to stay healthy."

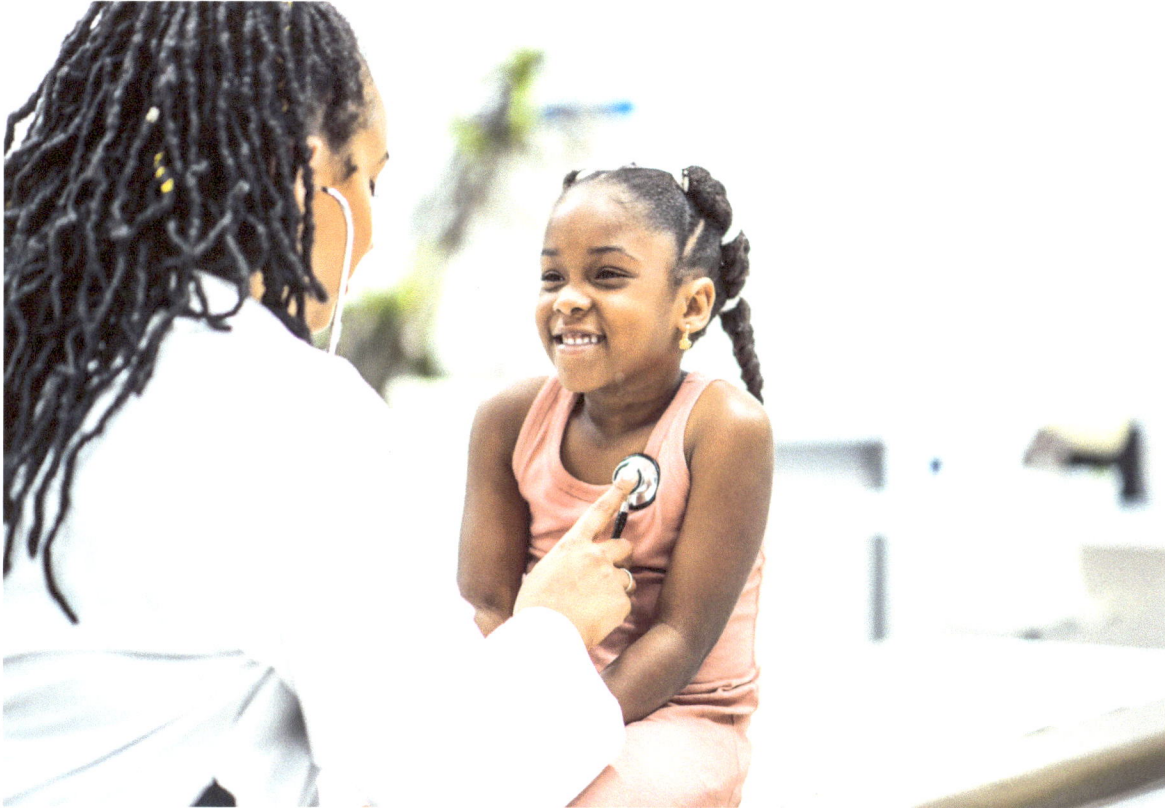

We go to the doctor for our annual check up
to stay healthy.

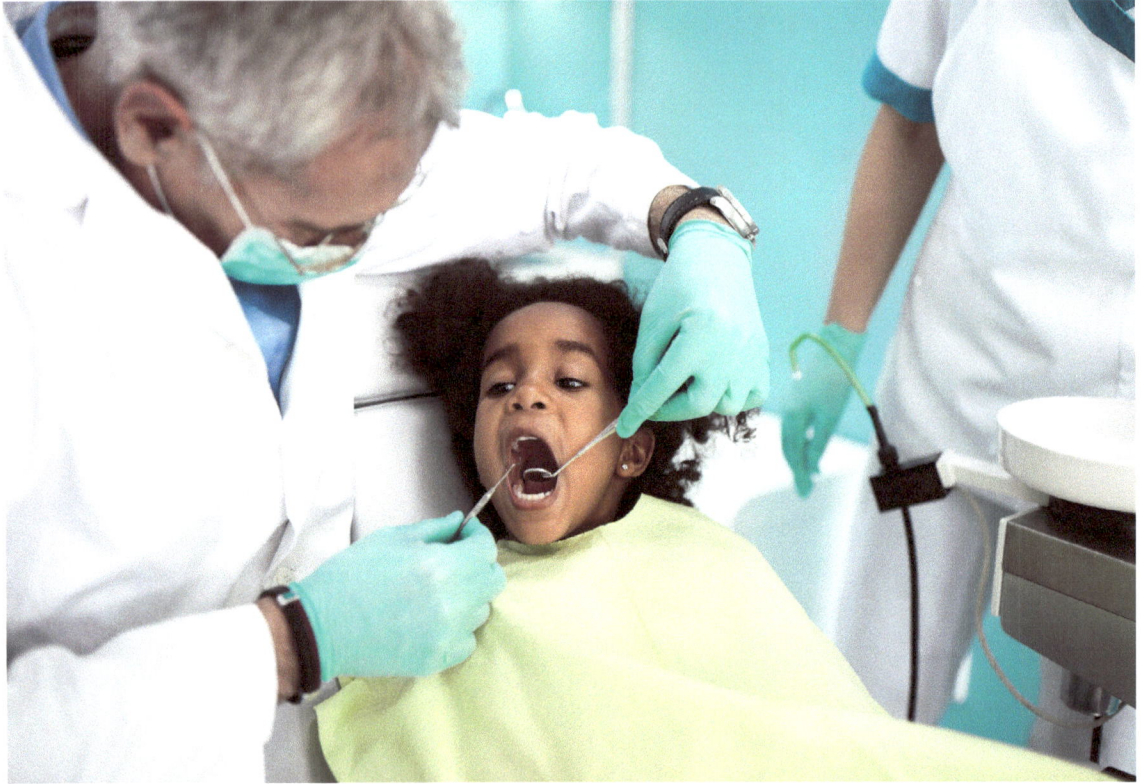

We have go to the dentist to stay healthy.

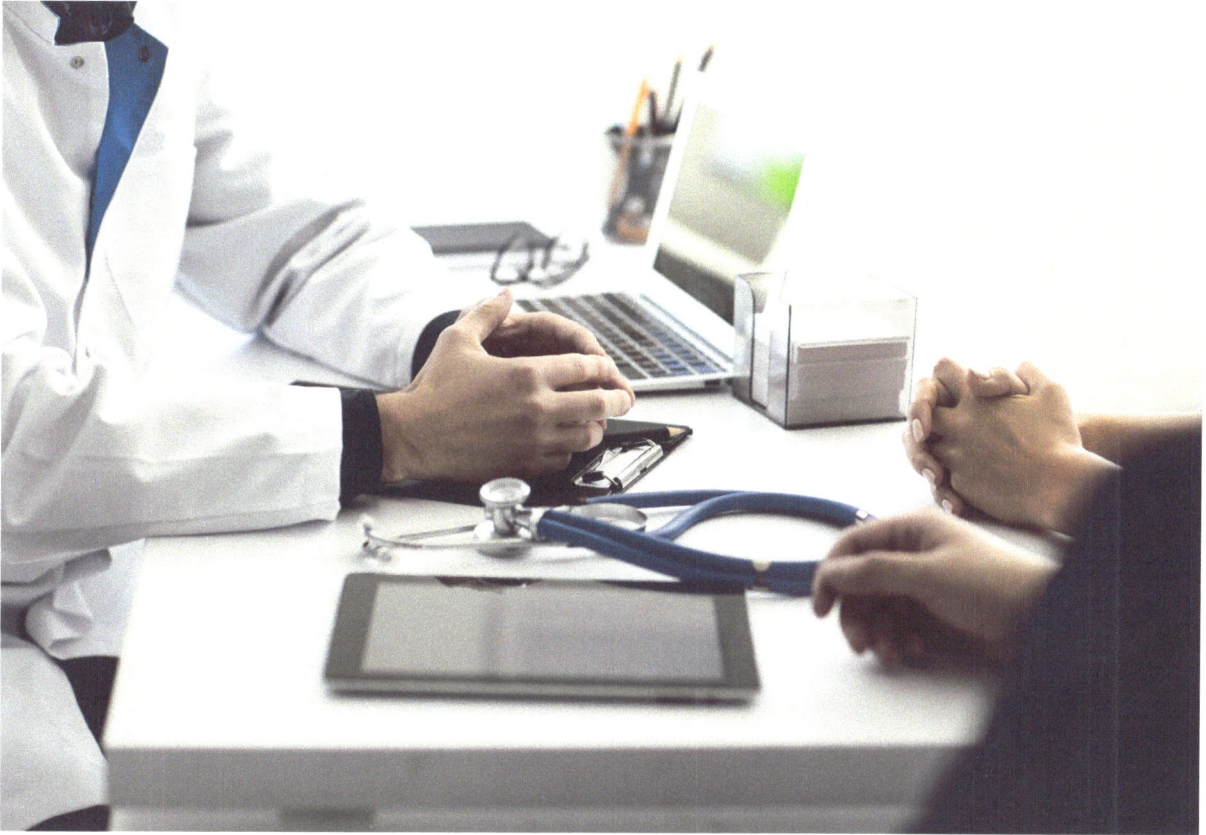

What about you?
Have you been to your doctor for your annual check up?

Draw and write about what you did at the doctor.

_____

_____

_____

_____

_____

_____

_____

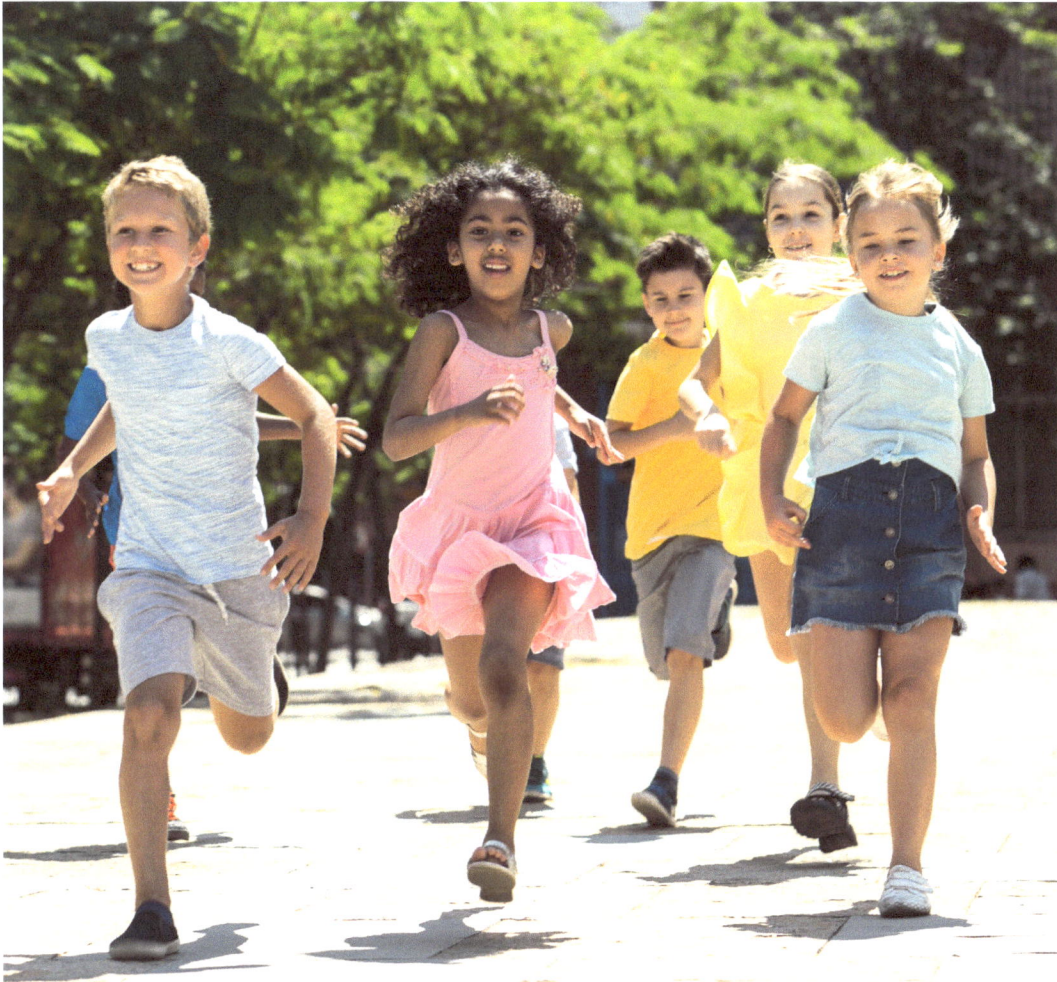

Some children say,
"Happiness keeps us healthy."

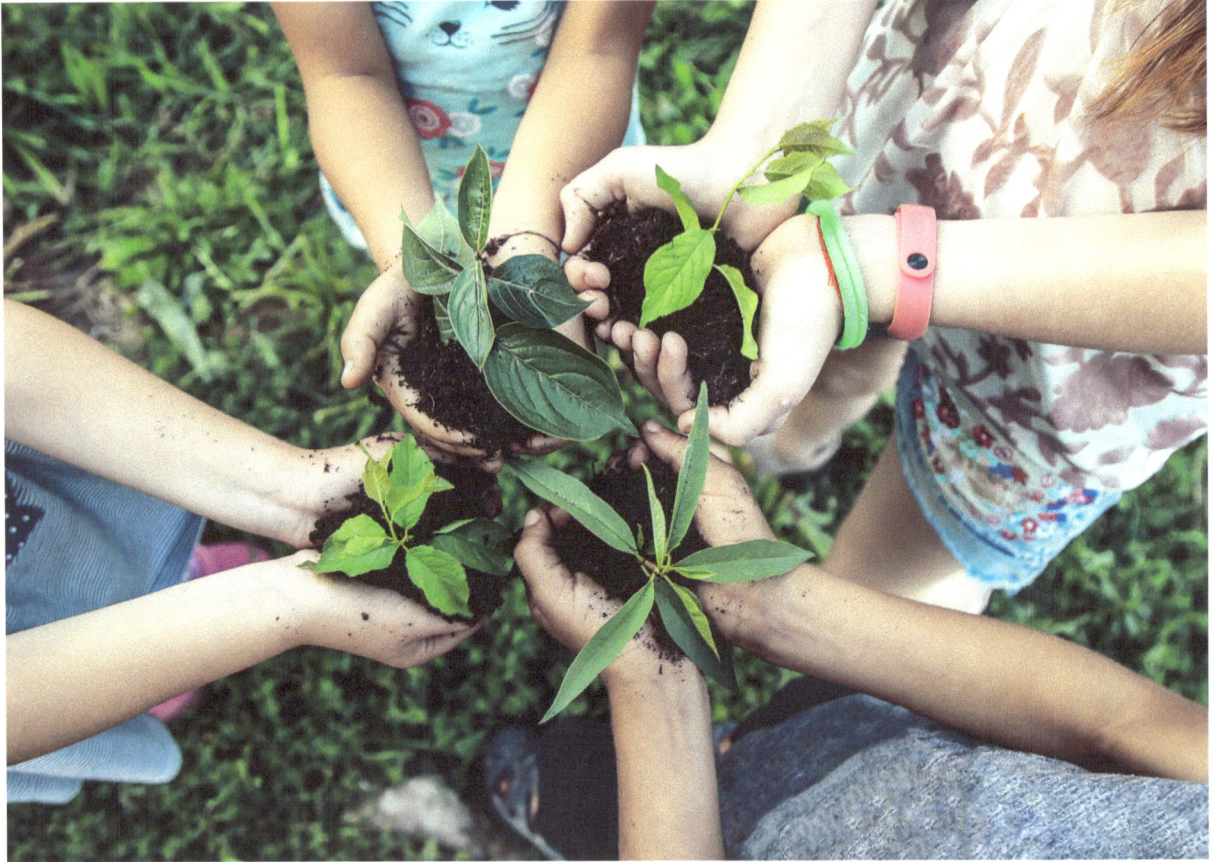

**Some children say,
"Gardening makes us happy."**

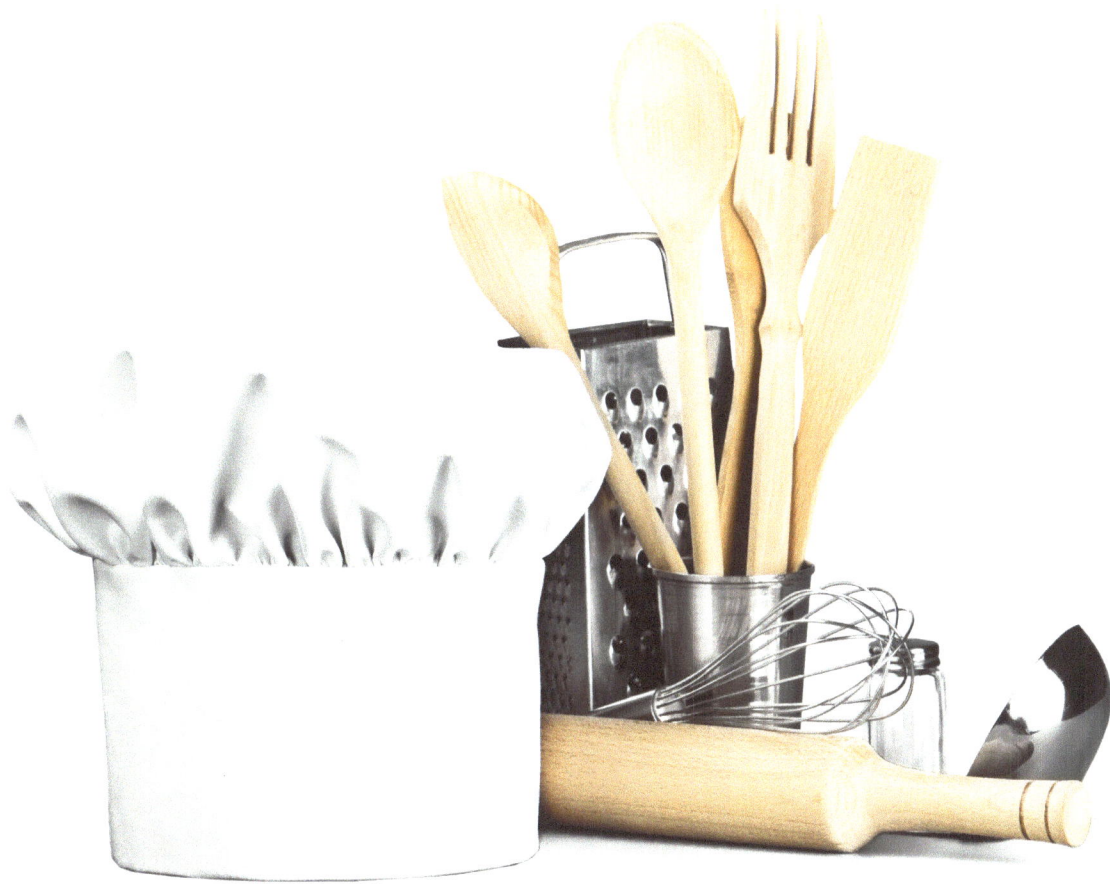

**Some children say,
"cooking makes us happy."**

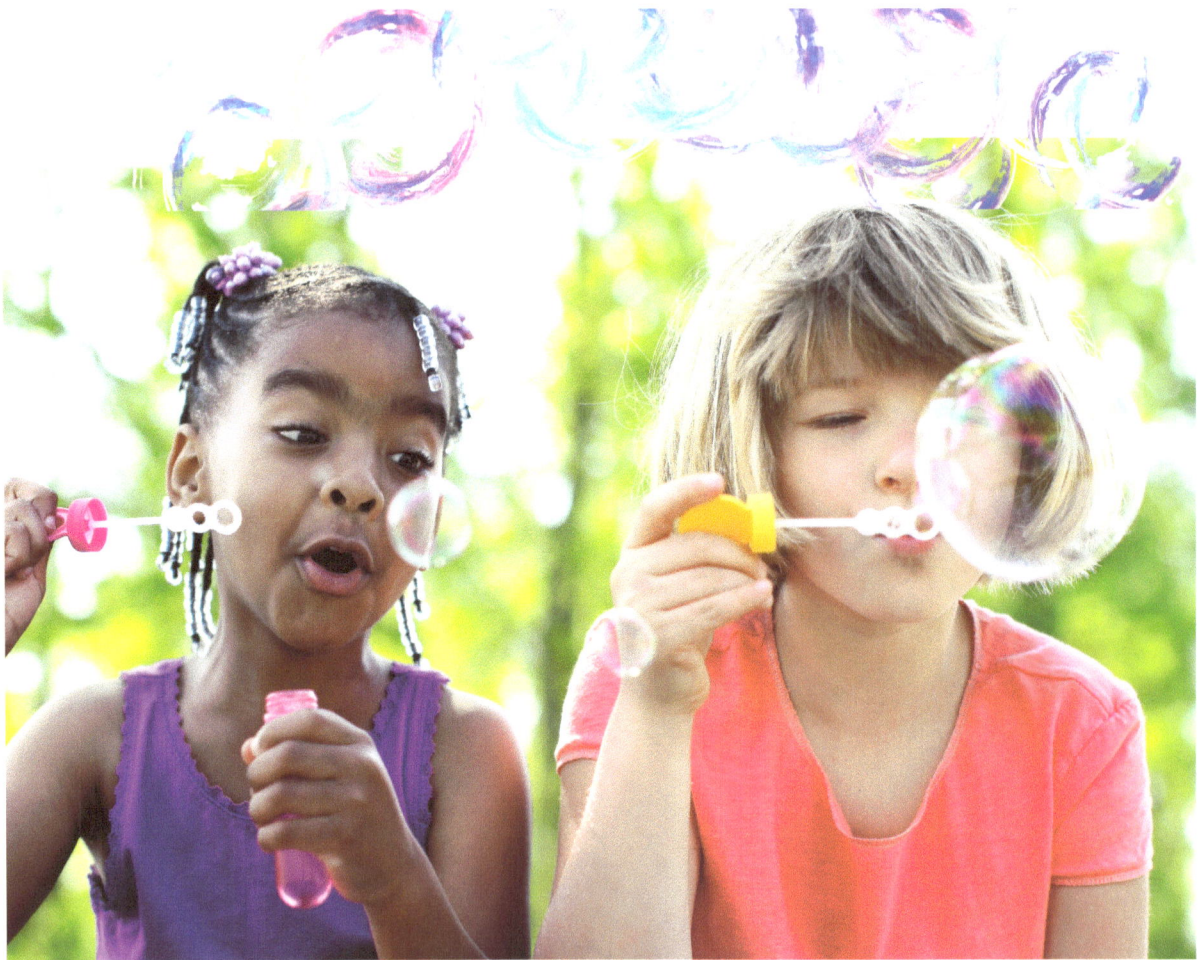

Some children say, "Playing with bubbles makes them happy."

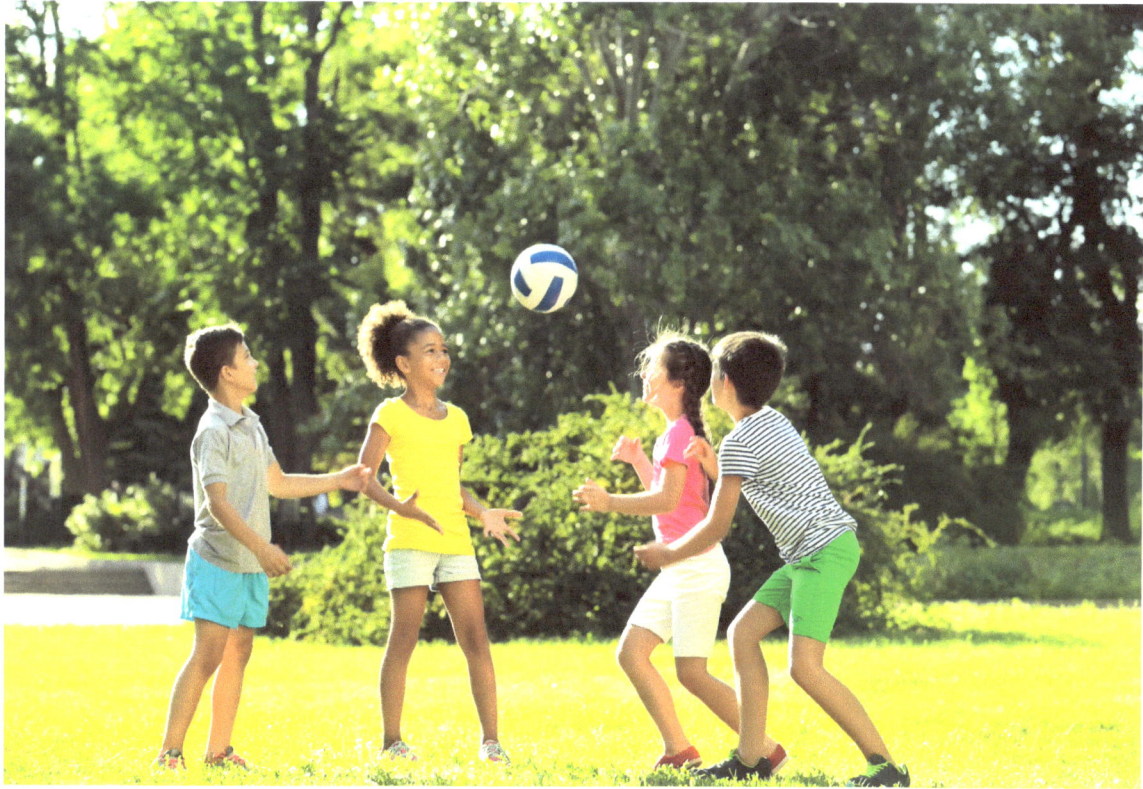

Some children says, "Playing with friends makes us happy."

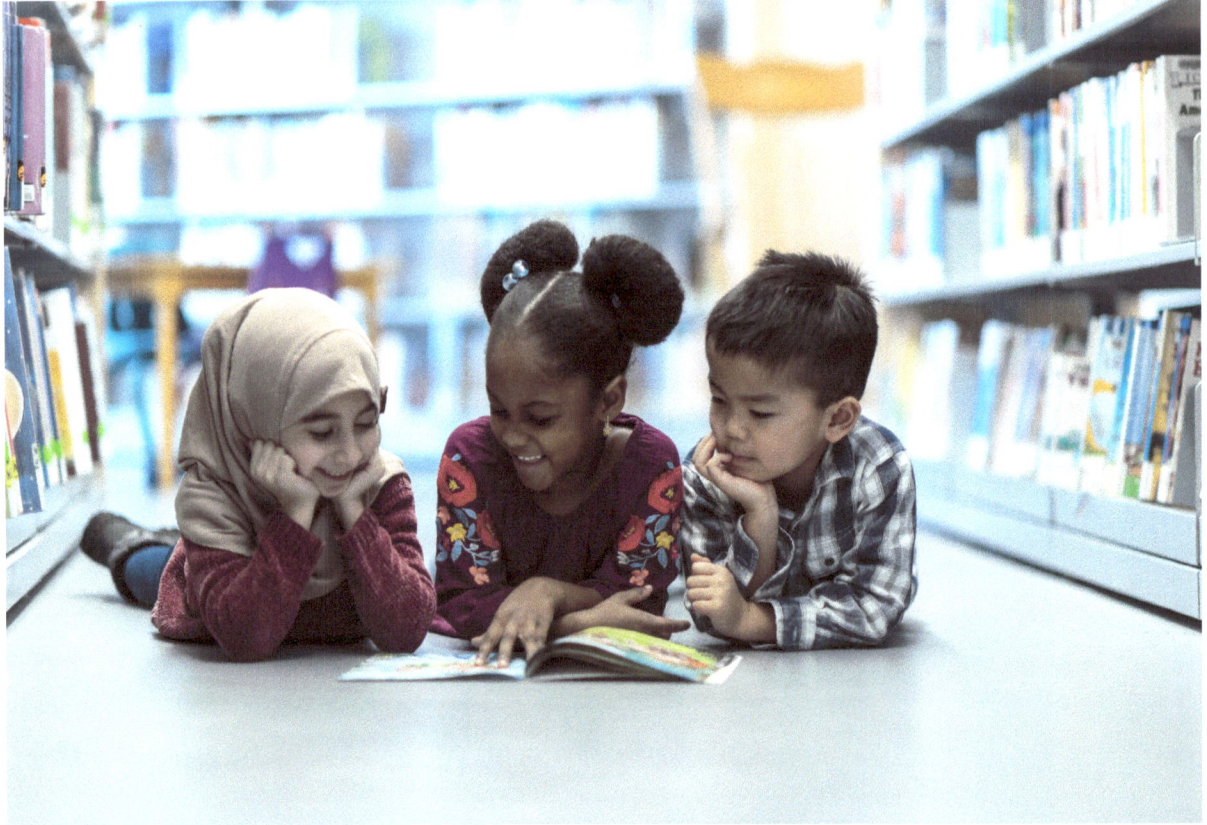

Some children say, "Reading books makes us happy."

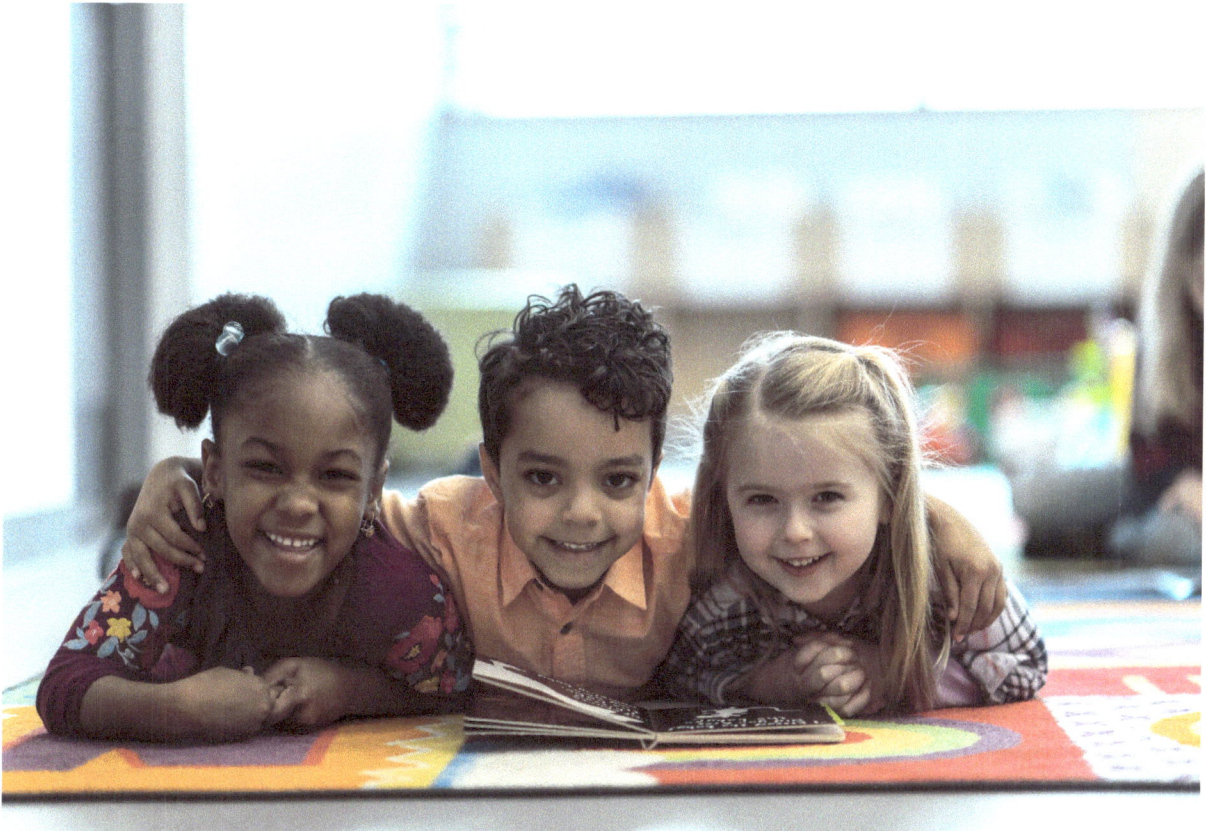

What makes you happy?

Look at Us!

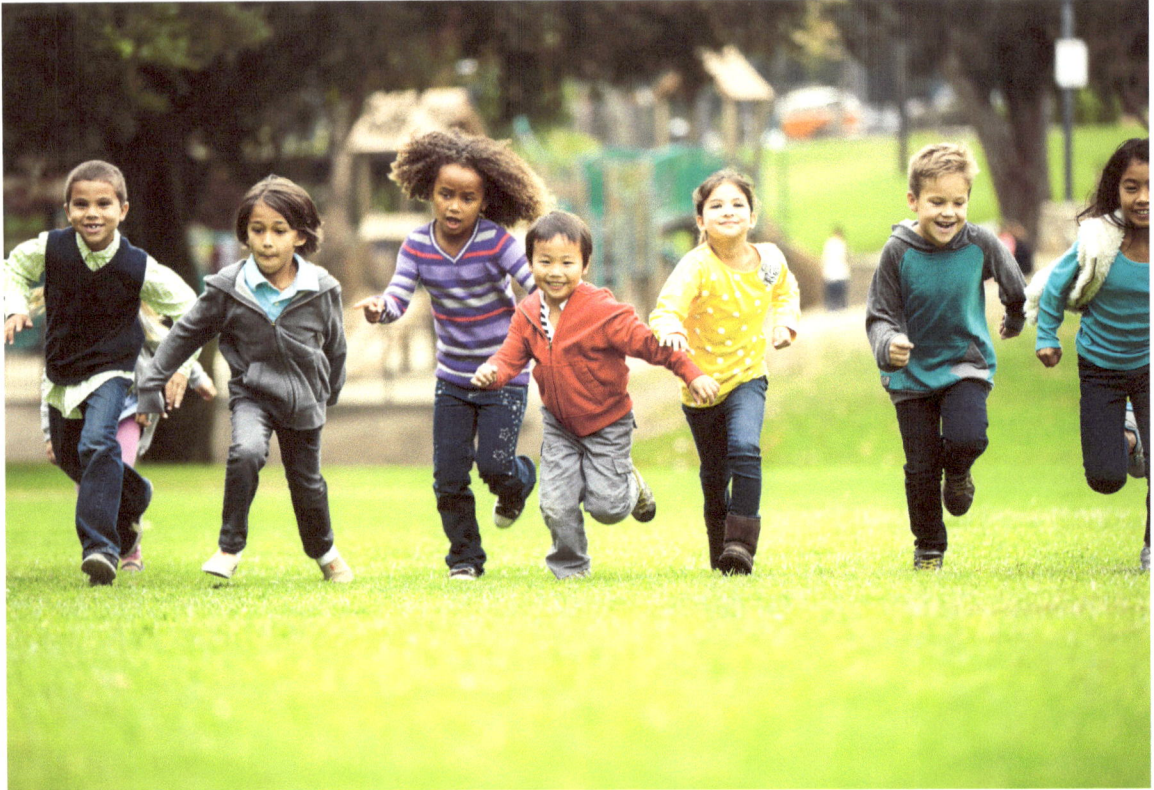

We are happy and healthy.

Adaptable Photos and Words

	sleep 	sleep
	shower 	shower
	soap 	soap
	water 	water

Adaptable Photos and Words

	wash hair	wash hair
	shampoo	shampoo
	comb	comb
	wash hands	wash hands

Adaptable Photos and Words

	soap	**soap**
	water	**water**
	brush teeth	**brush teeth**
	toothpaste	**toothpaste**

Adaptable Photos and Words

	toothbrush 	**toothbrush**
	floss 	**floss**
	mouthwash 	**mouthwash**
	food 	**food**

Adaptable Photos and Words

	meal	**meal**
	water	**water**
	plate	**plate**
	doctor	**doctor**

Adaptable Photos and Words

	dentist 	**dentist**
	gardening 	**gardening**
	cooking 	**cooking**
	bubbles 	**bubbles**

Adaptable Photos and Words

	playing	**playing**
	reading	**reading**
	children	**children**

www.ingramcontent.com/pod-product-compliance
Lightning Source LLC
Chambersburg PA
CBHW060859270326
41935CB00003B/39